NATURAL TREATMENT FOR FEMALE INFERTILITY

Blossoming Hope: Empowering Women Through A Natural Step-By-Step Guide To Becoming A Mother And Eradicating Infertility And Any Other Form Of Female Reproductive System Disorders.

MRS. VERA JACOB

Natural Treatment For Female Infertility

Copyright Notice. By Mrs. Vera Jacob

Contents

Introduction

Bringing new life into the world is a deeply human desire, one that has shaped the tapestry of our existence since time immemorial. The longing for parenthood is universal, a primal instinct that transcends culture, borders, and differences. It is a journey filled with hope, joy, and dreams of a family's future. However, for some, the path to parenthood is a road fraught with challenges, leading to a world of frustration, heartache, and uncertainty. The quest to conceive a child, which should be a natural and beautiful experience, becomes a daunting journey into the realm of infertility.

Today, millions of women have lost their homes, their culture, religion, beliefs, values, and relationships, some were even made housemaids and their housemaid takes their husbands from them. Some resulted in killing themselves because they couldn't withstand the insult (barren woman) from their mother-in-law, neighbors, and colleagues, some have lost hope of experiencing the joy of motherhood, some are scared of leaving their matrimonial home because they thought they could not conceive, some have suffered countless miscarriages, and some are suffering from fertility-related issues like; ovulation diseases, PCOS, POI, endometriosis, uterine fibroid, hormonal imbalance and lots more. In order to restore that confidence to the disgruntled woman and eradicate this nightmare called "Infertility" once and for all, Mrs. Jacob put together this guide titled "Natural Treatment for Female Infertility" as a simplified guide that will journey you through:

1. The alternative and holistic approaches to addressing infertility in women

2. The underlying causes of infertility

3. Provide you with insights on evidence-based information, and practical advice on natural treatments that would aid in enhancing fertility

4. Understanding how factors like environmental influences, nutrition, stress, and emotional well-being can impact fertility

5. Discussing lifestyle modifications

6. Different natural remedies and practices that can prevent, intervene, and treat infertility

7. Empowering women to make informed decisions and

take an active role in their fertility journey and a lot more.

Ultimately, this book is a testament to the resilience of the human spirit, the capacity for hope, and the ability to heal, both physically and emotionally. It is our hope that, armed with the knowledge and insights within these pages, you will find the strength to face the challenges of infertility.

As we embark on this journey together, remember that you are not defined by your challenges, but by your courage and determination. Let us begin the quest for natural solutions to infertility, with the belief that, in your future, a brighter and more fertile chapter awaits you. Do you still want to keep reading and be fertile, free from any form of infertility?

CHAPTER ONE
Understanding Infertility

Infertility is the inability to conceive after one year of unprotected intercourse, or six months for women over 35. It is a complex and emotionally challenging issue that affects individuals and couples from all walks of life. To effectively address infertility and explore natural treatment options, it's crucial to first understand its various facets.

The Role of Fertility

Fertility, the ability to conceive and bear children, is a delicate and intricate interplay of several factors, both in men and women. To grasp the concept of infertility, one must understand the fundamental components involved such as ovulation disorders, polycystic ovary syndrome, uterine fibroid, age-related factors, etc.

The Promise of Natural Treatments

When facing the challenges of infertility, many individuals

Natural Treatment For Female Infertility

and couples may explore various avenues to achieve their dreams of parenthood. While assisted reproductive technologies and medical interventions have made significant strides in helping people conceive, the promise of natural treatments cannot be overlooked. Natural treatments offer a holistic approach to infertility, emphasizing the importance of overall well-being and the body's innate capacity to heal and regenerate. Let's delve into the potential benefits and promise that natural treatments hold for those seeking to overcome infertility.

Natural treatments for infertility take a holistic approach, recognizing that fertility is not solely a physical issue but is intricately linked to your overall health and well-being. This holistic perspective views the body as a complex system of interconnected parts, and any imbalance or dysfunction in one area can affect fertility. By focusing on your overall wellness, you not only address the immediate challenges of infertility but also enhance your long-term health.

Fewer Side Effects

Compared to many medical treatments, natural remedies

often come with fewer side effects. This can be especially appealing to individuals who want to avoid or reduce the potential risks associated with pharmaceutical drugs or invasive medical procedures. Natural treatments typically involve dietary changes, lifestyle modifications, and herbal supplements, which are generally well-tolerated by the body.

Improved Emotional Well-Being

Infertility can take a significant toll on your emotional and psychological well-being. Natural treatments often include stress management techniques, mindfulness, and relaxation exercises that can help reduce the emotional burden of infertility. By nurturing your mental and emotional health, you may find it easier to navigate the emotional challenges that can arise during your fertility journey.

Enhanced Overall Health

Natural treatments not only aim to address infertility but also promote your overall health. By adopting a healthier lifestyle, you may reduce the risk of various chronic conditions and improve your quality of life. This can be particularly advantageous, as it creates a supportive foundation for your fertility journey and enhances your well-being even if conception does not occur immediately.

Personalized Approaches

Natural treatments often offer a more personalized approach to infertility. They take into account your unique health history, dietary preferences, and lifestyle, allowing you to tailor your treatment plan to your individual needs. This personalized approach can lead to more effective and sustainable results.

Complementary to Medical Interventions

Natural treatments need not be seen as an exclusive alternative to medical interventions. In many cases, they can be used in conjunction with conventional treatments to enhance their effectiveness. This synergy between natural and medical approaches can provide a more comprehensive

Natural Treatment For Female Infertility

strategy for addressing infertility.

As we journey through the pages of this book, you'll explore a wide range of natural treatments, from dietary and lifestyle changes to herbal remedies and alternative therapies. Our goal is to equip you with the knowledge and tools needed to make informed decisions about your fertility journey, and to offer hope and encouragement as you seek to fulfill your dreams of parenthood. While the path to overcoming infertility may be challenging, the promise of natural treatments offers a beacon of hope, emphasizing your body's incredible capacity to heal and nurture new life.

Causes of Infertility

Infertility is a complex issue, and its causes can vary extensively from person to person. Understanding the underpinning factors that contribute to gravidity is pivotal in order to address and overcome this gruelling condition. The causes of gravidity can be astronomically distributed into the following

Natural Treatment For Female Infertility

1. **Ovulation Diseases:** If you're experiencing difficulty conceiving as a result of uneven or distrait ovulation, know that you're not alone. This is a common issue faced by many women, but there are solutions available. Conditions like polycystic ovary syndrome (PCOS), hypothalamic dysfunction, and premature ovarian failure can all impact ovulation, but with the right medical intervention, these barriers can be overcome. Seeking professional assistance is the first step towards increasing your chances of conceiving. Remember, don't lose hope - you can achieve your goal of starting a family with the proper support and treatment.

2. **Polycystic Ovary Pattern (PCOS):** Polycystic Ovary Syndrome (PCOS) is a hormonal disorder that affects women and can cause irregular menstrual cycles and difficulties with ovulation.

3. **Endometriosis:** Endometriosis occurs when the tissue similar to the lining of the uterus grows outside the uterus, which can cause blockages in the fallopian tubes and affect fertility.

4. **Uterine Fibroids:** Non-cancerous growths in the uterus can impact fertility if they obstruct the fallopian tubes or intrude with embryo implantation.

5. **Age factors:** As women age, their egg quality and quantity decline, making conception more challenging.

6. **Hormonal Imbalance:** Hormonal imbalances, particularly related to the adrenal and pituitary glands, can also affect fertility.

Unexplained Infertility

Despite thorough medical evaluations, the exact cause of infertility in some cases remains unknown. In fact, coping with the physical and emotional challenges of infertility can prove to be a demanding and taxing experience

Numerous factors can have a detrimental impact on infertility women. Two of the most significant factors are smoking and alcohol consumption, which are known to have negative effects. Additionally, Exposure to environmental toxins, such as fungicides and chemicals, can harm fertility. It is essential to be mindful of these factors and to make necessary lifestyle changes to avoid potential harm. By doing so, one can manage and improve their fertility, leading to a healthier reproductive system and overall well-being. Diet and Exercise Poor nutrition, rotundity, and lack of physical exertion can contribute to gravidity. Stress High situations of stress can affect hormone products and disrupt the menstrual cycle, potentially leading to infertiliy. Weight Both being light and fat can impact fertility. It's important to note that gravidity is a multifaceted issue. numerous individualities and couples may have further than one factor contributing to their gravidity. relating the specific causes in your case is the first step toward getting an effective result. While medical interventions and supported reproductive technologies can give results, this book focuses on natural treatments and holistic approaches to address the underpinning causes of gravidity and ameliorate your chances of generality.

CHAPTER TWO
The Role Of Nutrition

Nutrition plays a critical role in fertility and reproductive health. The foods we eat provide the essential building blocks and energy necessary for the complex processes involved in conception. A well-balanced diet can support hormonal balance, ovulation, and sperm health, while also enhancing the overall health of both partners. Let's explore the key aspects of nutrition and its impact on fertility.

A Balanced Diet For Fertility

A well-rounded diet is essential for fertility. It should provide all the necessary macronutrients, including carbohydrates, proteins, and fats. These macronutrients offer energy and support the overall functioning of the body. Balancing your diet with the right mix of these macronutrients is crucial.

Micronutrients and Their Impact on Reproductive Health

Micronutrients, such as vitamins and minerals, are vital for fertility. They play specific roles in hormonal regulation, the development of healthy eggs and sperm, and embryo implantation. Some essential micronutrients for fertility include folate, vitamin D, vitamin E, and zinc.

The Role of Antioxidants in Fertility

Antioxidants play a crucial role in protecting the body from oxidative stress and damage caused by free radicals. These free radicals, which are highly reactive molecules, have the potential to cause cellular damage and contribute to the development of various health conditions, including cancer, heart disease, and neurodegenerative disorders. Antioxidants work by neutralizing the free radicals, thereby mitigating their harmful effects. Incorporating antioxidant-rich foods, such as fruits, vegetables, nuts, and seeds, into one's diet, is recommended to maintain optimal health and well-being. In the context of fertility, Antioxidant-rich fruits and vegetables protect eggs and sperm.

Superfoods for Fertility

Certain foods are recognized as fertility superfoods due to their nutritional content and potential to enhance reproductive health. These foods often contain a rich array of vitamins, minerals, and antioxidants. Examples of fertility-boosting superfoods include leafy greens, berries, fatty fish, and nuts.

Supplements and Fertility

In a situation where the infertility is as a result of deficiencies in some nutrients, dietary supplements can be recommended to address the fertility issue. Maintaining a healthy and well-balanced diet is crucial for ensuring fertility. However, sometimes our meals may not provide us with all the essential nutrients required for reproductive health. In such cases, supplements can be taken as an additional measure to complement the diet and help meet the crucial nutritional needs for fertility.

The Impact of Weight on Fertility

Maintaining a healthy weight is crucial for fertility since being underweight or overweight can disrupt hormonal balance and impact ovulation in women. Achieving a healthy weight through a balanced diet and regular exercise can significantly improve fertility.

Food to Avoid

Certain dietary choices can have a negative impact on fertility. These include excessive caffeine consumption, high alcohol intake, and the consumption of processed foods. It's important to recognize how these factors can affect reproductive health and make informed choices to reduce or eliminate their presence in your diet.

To support your fertility journey, dietary plans and meal ideas tailored for reproductive health can be beneficial. These plans provide guidance on incorporating fertility-boosting foods and making nutritious choices. Incorporating fertility-friendly meal ideas and recipes can help you prepare delicious and nutritious meals that can optimize your reproductive health and increase your chances of conception. By comprehending and effectively applying fundamental nutritional principles to your daily diet, you can effectively utilize the power of nutrition to enhance your fertility health. Proper nutrition can help regulate hormones, improve egg and sperm quality, promote healthy ovulation, and increase the likelihood of successful conception. Additionally, incorporating essential vitamins, minerals, and antioxidants into your diet can support a healthy pregnancy and reduce the risk of complications. Therefore, it is vital to understand and implement these principles into your daily eating habits to optimize your fertility health and increase your chances of conceiving. The role of nutrition in fertility is a fundamental aspect of a holistic approach to addressing infertility, recognizing that the food you eat not only nourishes your body but also nurtures the potential for new life.

CHAPTER THREE
Lifestyle Modifications

Lifestyle plays a significant role in fertility, and making positive changes can enhance your chances of conceiving. Whether you're struggling with infertility or simply looking to optimize your reproductive health, the following lifestyle modifications can make a difference:

Stress Management

Chronic stress can disrupt the delicate hormonal balance necessary for fertility. Reducing stress can have a significant impact on your well-being and potentially improve your chances of conceiving. Managing stress can be crucial when dealing with infertility.

Chronic stress can lead to the release of stress hormones like cortisol, which can disrupt the hormonal balance in the body. This hormonal imbalance may affect the menstrual cycle and ovulation in women. Managing stress can help normalize hormone levels.

Stress management tactics, such as relaxation exercises,

meditation, can improve your overall health, which in turn can have a positive impact on your reproductive health.

For individuals undergoing fertility treatments, stress management techniques can help reduce anxiety and improve the overall experience. Lower stress levels may enhance the effectiveness of treatments such as in vitro fertilization (IVF).

Stress management can also help improve communication between partners. Coping with infertility can be emotionally challenging, and practicing effective communication and support can strengthen the relationship during this difficult time.

While stress management can be a useful part of a comprehensive approach to dealing with infertility, it should be viewed as one piece of the puzzle, along with medical interventions and lifestyle adjustments.

Exercise and Fertility

Regular physical activity is important for overall health, but excessive or intense exercise can sometimes negatively impact fertility, especially in women. Engaging in moderate exercise can support weight management and overall well-being, which are essential for fertility.

Here are ways in which exercise may positively impact fertility:

1. **Maintaining a Healthy Weight**: Obesity or being underweight can affect hormonal balance and disrupt the menstrual cycle, leading to fertility issues. Regular exercise, combined with a balanced diet, can help regulate weight and improve overall health.

2. **Balancing Hormones:** Exercise can help regulate hormones, such as insulin and cortisol, which may impact fertility. High levels of stress and insulin resistance can disrupt reproductive hormones.

3. **Improving Circulation:** Exercise increases blood flow throughout the body, including the pelvic region, which is important for reproductive health. Improved circulation can enhance the delivery of oxygen and nutrients to reproductive organs.

4. **Managing Stress:** Chronic stress can negatively affect fertility. Exercise is a natural stress reliever, as

it prompts the release of endorphins, which can help improve mood and reduce stress levels.

5. **Enhancing Mental Health:** Mental health is closely linked to reproductive health. Exercise has been shown to reduce symptoms of anxiety and depression, which can indirectly benefit fertility.

6. **Regulating Menstrual Cycle:** Regular physical activity may help regulate the menstrual cycle, making it more predictable and increasing the chances of conception. It's important to note that while moderate exercise is generally beneficial, excessive and intense exercise may have negative effects on fertility in some cases. Striking a balance and adopting a moderate exercise routine is key.

Sleep and Fertility

Consistent, restorative sleep is vital for reproductive health. Sleep disturbances and insufficient sleep can disrupt the body's hormonal rhythms, affecting ovulation and sperm production. Creating a healthy sleep routine and addressing sleep issues can positively impact fertility.

Smoking and Alcohol Intake

Both smoking and too much intake of alcohol are known to have detrimental effects on fertility. They can disrupt the menstrual cycle, and increase the risk of pregnancy complications. Quitting smoking and reducing alcohol intake are important steps in improving fertility.

Environmental Toxins

Exposure to environmental toxins, such as pesticides, pollutants, and certain chemicals, can interfere with fertility. Reducing exposure to these toxins, both at home and in the workplace, is essential.

By making these lifestyle modifications, you can create an environment that is conducive to fertility and overall well-being. These changes not only increase your chances of conception but also contribute to a healthier, more balanced lifestyle. Embracing a holistic approach that combines nutrition, lifestyle modifications, and other natural treatments can be a powerful strategy for addressing infertility and improving your chances of achieving your dream of parenthood.

CHAPTER FOUR
Herbal Remedies And Alternative Therapies
Traditional Herbal Remedies

Traditional herbal remedies have been used for centuries across various cultures to address health concerns, including those related to fertility. Some herbs are believed to have properties that may support reproductive health. However, it's crucial to approach herbal remedies with caution, as not all herbs are safe, and their efficacy is not always scientifically proven. Consultation with a healthcare professional is recommended before incorporating herbal remedies into your fertility journey.

Acupuncture

Some studies suggest that acupuncture may positively impact fertility by promoting blood flow to the reproductive organs, balancing hormones, and reducing stress. While research is ongoing, many individuals exploring alternative therapies for fertility choose to include acupuncture in their treatment plans.

Chiropractic Care

Some proponents believe that chiropractic adjustments can help optimize the nervous system, leading to improved reproductive function. However, evidence supporting chiropractic care specifically for fertility is limited, and consultation with a healthcare provider is advised.

Homeopathy

Homeopathy is a holistic system of medicine based on the principle of "like cures like." Tiny amounts of natural substances that would produce symptoms in a healthy person are used to stimulate healing in someone experiencing similar symptoms. While some individuals turn to homeopathy for fertility support, scientific evidence supporting its effectiveness is scarce. As with any alternative therapy, consult with a healthcare professional before use.

Naturopathy

Naturopathy emphasizes natural healing modalities and

lifestyle interventions to promote overall well-being. Naturopathic approaches to fertility may include dietary changes, nutritional supplements, and herbal remedies. A naturopathic doctor can provide personalized guidance based on an individual's health history and needs.

Aromatherapy

Aromatherapy involves the use of essential oils for therapeutic purposes. While aromatherapy may be employed to reduce stress and promote relaxation, limited scientific evidence supports its direct impact on fertility. Caution is advised when using essential oils, especially during pregnancy, and consultation with a healthcare professional is recommended.

Ayurveda

Ayurveda, an ancient system of medicine from India, considers balance in the body's doshas (bio energies) as essential for overall health. Ayurvedic practices for fertility may include dietary changes, herbal supplements, and lifestyle recommendations. Consulting with an Ayurvedic practitioner can provide personalized guidance aligned with Ayurvedic principles.

It's crucial to approach alternative therapies with an open mind while also considering scientific evidence and consulting with healthcare professionals. Integrating alternative therapies into a comprehensive fertility plan should be done in collaboration with medical experts to ensure safety and efficacy.

CHAPTER FIVE
Managing Hormonal Imbalances

Managing hormonal imbalances involves a multifaceted approach that includes lifestyle changes, dietary modifications, stress management, and, in some cases, medical interventions. Hormones play a crucial role in various bodily functions, and an imbalance can affect overall health and well-being. Here are some general strategies for managing hormonal imbalances:

Regular Exercise: Engage in regular physical activity to help regulate hormones, reduce stress, and maintain a healthy weight.

Lifestyle Management

Adequate Sleep: Ensure you get sufficient, quality sleep each night, as lack of sleep can disrupt hormonal balance.

Stress Management: Practice stress-reducing techniques such as meditation, deep breathing exercises, yoga, or mindfulness to regulate cortisol levels.

Limiting Exposure to Endocrine Disruptors:

Natural Treatment For Female Infertility

Minimize exposure to environmental toxins and endocrine disruptors found in certain plastics, pesticides, and household products.

Dietary Modifications

Omega-3 Fatty Acids: Include sources of omega-3 fatty acids, such as fatty fish, flaxseeds, and walnuts, which can help support hormonal balance.

Fiber-Rich Foods: Increase fiber intake from whole grains, fruits, and vegetables to support digestive health and hormone metabolism.

Healthy Fats: Include sources of healthy fats, such as avocados, olive oil, and nuts, which are essential for hormone production.

Limit Caffeine and Alcohol: Reduce consumption of caffeine and alcohol, as excessive intake can disrupt hormonal balance.

Medical Interventions

Consultation with Healthcare Professionals: If you suspect

Natural Treatment For Female Infertility

a hormonal imbalance, consult with a healthcare professional. They can conduct tests to identify specific hormonal imbalances and recommend appropriate interventions.

Hormone Replacement Therapy (HRT): In cases of severe hormonal imbalances, hormone replacement therapy may be prescribed under the guidance of a healthcare provider.

Medications: Certain medications may be prescribed to regulate specific hormones. This could include medications for thyroid disorders, insulin resistance, or other hormonal conditions.

Herbal Remedies and Supplements

Consult an Herbalist or Naturopath: Some herbs and supplements are believed to support hormonal balance. Consult an herbalist or a naturopath to help with personalizing the herbs.

Vitamins and Minerals: Ensure adequate intake of essential vitamins and minerals, such as vitamin D, zinc, and magnesium, which play a role in hormonal health.

Natural Treatment For Female Infertility

Adaptogenic Herbs: Consider adaptogenic herbs like ashwagandha or Rhodiola, which are thought to help the body adapt to stress and support hormone balance.

It's essential to note that individual needs vary, and what works for one person may not work for another. It's advisable to work with healthcare professionals, including endocrinologists, nutritionists, and other specialists, to create a comprehensive and personalized plan.

Balancing Female Hormones

It is very important that you maintain a healthy weight through consistent exercise and a balanced diet.

Nutrient-Rich Diet: Consume a diet rich in fruits, vegetables, whole grains, and lean proteins. Include foods with omega-3 fatty acids, like fatty fish and flaxseeds, which can support hormone production.

Manage Blood Sugar Levels: Opt for complex carbohydrates and balance meals to prevent spikes and crashes in blood sugar levels. This helps regulate insulin, a key hormone.

Consistent Exercise: Engaging oneself with a regular

Natural Treatment For Female Infertility

physical exercise like aerobic exercises and any other form of strength training can help regulate estrogen levels and improve overall hormonal balance.

Adequate Sleep: Ensure you get enough quality sleep, as insufficient sleep can disrupt the balance of hormones such as estrogen, progesterone, and cortisol.

Manage Stress: Practice stress-reducing techniques such as yoga, meditation, and deep breathing. Chronic stress can negatively impact female hormones.

Limit Caffeine and Alcohol: Moderate your intake of caffeine and alcohol, as excessive consumption can affect hormonal balance, including estrogen levels.

Consider Hormonal Birth Control: In some cases, hormonal birth control methods may be used to regulate menstrual cycles and hormone levels.

The Role of Stress Hormones

Stress hormones play a crucial role in the body's response to stress, helping to prepare the body to face challenges or threats. The primary stress hormones include cortisol and adrenaline (also known as epinephrine). While these hormones are essential for survival in acute stress situations, chronic or prolonged stress can lead to imbalances, impacting physical and mental health.

Role of Stress Hormones

Cortisol: Release in Response to Stress: Cortisol is often referred to as the "stress hormone" and is released by the adrenal glands in response to stress. It helps the body respond to a perceived threat by increasing alertness and energy.

Blood Sugar Regulation: Cortisol plays a key role in regulating blood sugar levels. It promotes the release of glucose into the bloodstream, providing the body with a quick source of energy.

Immune Function: Cortisol also has anti-inflammatory properties and plays a role in regulating the immune system's response to inflammation.

Daily Rhythm (Circadian Rhythm): Cortisol follows a natural daily rhythm, typically peaking in the early morning and reaching its lowest levels in the evening and during sleep.

Adrenaline (Epinephrine): Immediate Response to Stress: Adrenaline is released rapidly in response to acute stress. It prepares the body for a "fight or flight" response by increasing heart rate, dilating airways, and redirecting blood flow to muscles.

Short-Term Energy Boost: Adrenaline mobilizes energy stores, providing a quick burst of energy to deal with immediate threats.

Impact of Chronic Stress

Disruption of Hormonal Balance: Prolonged stress can lead to an imbalance in cortisol levels, disrupting the normal circadian rhythm. This can result in symptoms such as fatigue, insomnia, or difficulty concentrating.

Impact on Immune Function: Chronic stress may suppress the immune system, making the body more susceptible to infections and illnesses.

Metabolic Effects: Elevated cortisol levels over the long term can contribute to metabolic disturbances, including

Natural Treatment For Female Infertility

insulin resistance and increased abdominal fat.

Cardiovascular Effects: Chronic stress is associated with an increased risk of cardiovascular problems, including high blood pressure and heart disease.

Mental Health Impact: Prolonged stress can contribute to mental health issues, such as anxiety and depression.

Reproductive Effects: Chronic stress may impact reproductive hormones, leading to irregular menstrual cycles in women and potential fertility issues.

Managing Stress Hormones

Stress Management Techniques: Practice stress-reducing activities such as meditation, deep breathing exercises, yoga, or mindfulness to help manage the body's stress response.

Regular Exercise: Engage in regular physical activity, which can help regulate stress hormones and promote overall well-being.

Adequate Sleep: Ensure sufficient, quality sleep, as sleep is crucial for the regulation of stress hormones and overall

Natural Treatment For Female Infertility
health.

Healthy Lifestyle: Adopt a balanced and healthy lifestyle, including a nutritious diet, regular exercise, and sufficient rest.

Social Support: Maintain strong social connections and seek support from friends, family, or professionals when needed.

Mindfulness Practices: Practices such as mindfulness meditation can be effective in reducing stress and promoting emotional well-being.

If stress is significantly impacting your health, consider seeking guidance from healthcare professionals or mental health specialists.

Herbal Medicine for Hormonal Balance

While herbal medicines are often suggested for hormone balance, it's important to approach them with caution and consult with a healthcare professional before incorporating them into your routine. The effectiveness of herbal remedies can vary, and some may interact with medications or have side effects. Here are several herbs that are commonly

Natural Treatment For Female Infertility

associated with supporting hormone balance:

Chasteberry (Vitex): Often used to alleviate symptoms associated with hormonal imbalances in women, including irregular menstrual cycles, premenstrual syndrome (PMS), and menopausal symptoms. It is thought to influence the balance of reproductive hormones, especially estrogen and progesterone.

Black Cohosh: Commonly used to address menopausal symptoms, black cohosh may help regulate estrogen levels and alleviate hot flashes and mood swings.

Dong Quai: A traditional Chinese herb believed to support women's reproductive health and balance hormones. It is often used to regulate menstrual cycles and alleviate menstrual cramps.

Red Clover: this is a herbal remedy that contains isoflavones that can function exactly like estrogen. Red clover is sometimes used to alleviate menopausal symptoms and support hormonal balance.

Maca Root: Known as an adaptogenic herb, maca root is believed to help balance hormones in both men and women.

Natural Treatment For Female Infertility

It is thought to influence the endocrine system and support reproductive health.

Ashwagandha: An adaptogenic herb that may help the body adapt to stress. It is believed to have a balancing effect on cortisol, the stress hormone, and may support overall hormonal balance.

Licorice Root: May help regulate cortisol levels and support adrenal function. However, long-term or excessive use of licorice root should be approached cautiously due to potential side effects.

Wild Yam: Contains compounds that are precursors to progesterone. While it doesn't directly increase progesterone levels, it is sometimes used to support hormonal balance.

Always consult with a healthcare professional, especially if you have underlying health conditions, are taking medications, or are pregnant or breastfeeding. Herbal remedies should be used under supervision to ensure safety and efficacy.

CHAPTER SIX
Natural Approaches To Improve Egg Quality
Introduction:

The quality of eggs is crucial for successful conception and a healthy pregnancy. While various factors can influence reproductive health, incorporating natural approaches to enhance egg quality may positively impact fertility outcomes. This chapter explores lifestyle changes, dietary interventions, and holistic practices that individuals and couples can consider to optimize egg quality.

Enhancing Egg Quality

Enhancing egg quality is crucial for successful conception and a healthy pregnancy. While the quality of eggs can be influenced by various factors, there are natural approaches that individuals can consider to optimize egg health. It's important to note that these strategies should be discussed with a healthcare professional, especially for those actively trying to conceive. Here are some natural approaches to enhance egg quality:

1. Nutrient-Rich Diet: Include a variety of fruits,

vegetables, whole grains, lean proteins, and healthy fats to provide essential nutrients that support egg development.

2. Antioxidant-Rich Foods: Incorporate foods high in antioxidants, such as berries, nuts, seeds, and leafy greens. Antioxidants help protect eggs from oxidative stress, which can negatively impact egg quality.

3. Omega-3 Fatty Acids: Include sources of omega-3 fatty acids, such as fatty fish, chia seeds, and flaxseeds, in your diet. Omega-3s contribute to overall reproductive health and may support egg quality.

4. Coenzyme Q10 (CoQ10) Supplementation: Some studies suggest that CoQ10 supplementation may improve egg quality, especially in women of advanced maternal age.

5. Folic Acid and B Vitamins: Ensure adequate intake of folic acid and B vitamins, which are essential for DNA synthesis and repair. These nutrients are crucial for healthy egg development.

6. Vitamin D: Maintain optimal levels of vitamin D, as

it plays a role in reproductive health. Sun exposure and vitamin D-rich foods or supplements can contribute to sufficient levels.

7. Regular Exercise: Engage in moderate, regular exercise to support overall health, improve blood flow, and enhance hormonal balance, all of which contribute to better egg quality.

Lifestyle Changes for Better Fertility

Making positive lifestyle changes can significantly impact fertility for both men and women. These changes promote overall health and create an environment conducive to successful conception. Here are lifestyle modifications for better fertility:

1. Maintain a Healthy Weight: Achieve and maintain a healthy weight through a balanced diet and regular exercise.

2. Regular Exercise: Engage in regular physical activity. Moderate exercise helps regulate hormones and contributes to overall well-being. However, excessive exercise may have negative effects, so moderation is

key.

3. Balanced Diet: Consume a nutrient-rich diet that includes fruits, vegetables, whole grains, lean proteins, and healthy fats. Proper nutrition supports hormonal balance and reproductive health.

4. Adequate Sleep: Prioritize sufficient, quality sleep. Lack of sleep can disrupt hormonal balance, including reproductive hormones.

5. Manage Stress: Practice stress-reducing techniques such as meditation, deep breathing, yoga, or mindfulness. Chronic stress can impact fertility.

6. Quit Smoking: Smoking has been linked to reduced fertility in women. Quitting smoking is beneficial for overall health and reproductive well-being.

7. Avoid Excessive Heat: Avoid prolonged exposure to high temperatures, such as hot tubs and saunas, as elevated body temperature can affect egg quality.

8. Regular Menstrual Cycle Tracking: Track your menstrual cycle to understand your fertile window and increase the chances of conception.

9. Preconception Checkup: Schedule a preconception

> checkup with a healthcare provider to address any underlying health issues and receive guidance on optimizing fertility.

Remember that fertility is a complex interplay of various factors, and individual responses may vary. If there are concerns about fertility, seeking guidance from a healthcare professional or a fertility specialist is advisable. They can provide personalized advice based on individual circumstances and may recommend further evaluation if needed.

Fertility-Boosting Mindset Introduction

A fertility-boosting mindset is a powerful and often underestimated aspect of the journey toward conception. This chapter explores the transformative influence of positivity, introduces mind-body techniques, and delves into the efficacy of visualization and affirmations in fostering a conducive mental environment for fertility.

The Power of Positivity

Positivity is a transformative force that extends far beyond mere emotional well-being; it holds the potential to influence various aspects of our lives, including the intricate journey of fertility. In this section, we explore the profound impact of cultivating a positive mindset on the fertility process.

Understanding Positivity and Fertility

Stress and Fertility: Stress can significantly impact fertility, affecting both men and women. Understanding the complex relationship between stress and fertility is crucial for individuals and couples navigating the journey toward conception. Here's an exploration of the ways in which stress can influence fertility:

1. Hormonal Disruption: Chronic stress triggers the release of cortisol, a hormone associated with the body's "fight or flight" response. Elevated cortisol levels can disrupt the balance of reproductive hormones, including those responsible for ovulation and sperm production.

2. Menstrual Irregularities: Stress can lead to irregular menstrual cycles in women. It may cause anovulation (lack of ovulation) or affect the regularity of the menstrual cycle, making it challenging to predict fertile days.

3. Impact on Ovulation: For women trying to conceive, stress might interfere with the process of ovulation. An irregular ovulation cycle can reduce the opportunities for conception.

4. Changes in Libido: Stress can lead to a decrease in libido, impacting the frequency of intercourse. Reduced sexual activity can, in turn, lower the chances of conception.

5. Delayed Time to Pregnancy: Couples experiencing high levels of stress may take longer to achieve pregnancy compared to those with lower stress levels. The longer time to conception could be a result of hormonal imbalances and other stress-related factors.

6. Assisted Reproductive Technologies (ART) Outcomes: Stress may influence the outcomes of

assisted reproductive technologies (ART) such as in vitro fertilization (IVF). Some studies suggest that high stress levels during IVF treatment may be associated with lower success rates.

7. Psychological Impact: The emotional toll of fertility struggles can contribute to stress. The pressure to conceive, anxiety about fertility treatments, and the uncertainty of the outcome can create a cycle of stress that further hampers fertility.

8. Coping Mechanisms: Individuals may employ unhealthy coping mechanisms to deal with stress, such as smoking, excessive alcohol consumption, or poor dietary habits, which can have negative effects on fertility.

Stress-Reducing Strategies

Strategy: Mindful breathing description: Mindful breathing, also known as deep or diaphragmatic breathing, is a simple yet powerful stress-reducing technique. It involves consciously directing your breath to promote relaxation and reduce the physiological and psychological effects of stress.

How to Practice Stress Reducing Strategies

1. Find a Quiet Space

2. Sit or lie in a comfortable position. If sitting, ensure your back is straight, and your shoulders are relaxed.

3. Focus on Your Breath

4. Close your eyes if it feels comfortable.

5. Inhale Slowly and Deeply

6. Inhale deeply, feel the breath filling your lungs, and let your abdomen rise.

7. Exhale Slowly and Completely

8. As you inhale and exhale, count each breath cycle. For example, inhale for a count of four, hold for a count of two, and exhale for a count of six.

9. Keep your focus on your breath.

10. Practice mindful breathing for a few minutes, gradually extending the duration as you become more comfortable with the technique.

Benefits of Stress Reduction

1. Stress Reduction: Mindful breathing activates the body's relaxation response, reducing stress and promoting a sense of calm.

2. Anxiety Management: It is effective in managing anxiety by bringing attention to the present moment.

3. Lowered Blood Pressure: Deep breathing can contribute to lower blood pressure, especially when practiced consistently.

When to Use Stress Reduction Technique?

1. Use this technique during moments of heightened stress or anxiety.

2. Practice it regularly as part of a daily routine to build resilience to stress over time.

3. Incorporate mindful breathing into activities such as meditation or yoga for a more holistic approach to stress reduction.

Note: Individual responses to stress-reducing strategies may vary. If stress persists or worsens, it's advisable to consult with a healthcare professional or a mental health practitioner for personalized guidance and support.

Holistic Well-Being:

Fertility is not solely a physical process; it is deeply intertwined with mental and emotional aspects. A holistic approach to well-being is essential in understanding the intricate connection between mental and physical health in the context of fertility.

What Are the Mind-Body Techniques?

The mind body techniques are:

1. **Visualization and Affirmations:** Body-mind techniques, also known as mind-body techniques, involve practices that acknowledge the interconnectedness of the body and mind. These approaches recognize the influence of mental and emotional well-being on physical health and vice versa. Here are several body-mind techniques that promote holistic wellness:

   i. **Mindfulness Meditation:** Mindfulness

> meditation involves cultivating awareness of the present moment without judgment. It often includes focusing on the breath, sensations, or a specific point of focus.
>
> **ii.** **Benefits:** Reduces stress, enhances self-awareness, improves concentration, and promotes emotional well-being.

2. **Yoga:** Emphasizes the mind-body connection and aims to promote flexibility, strength, and inner peace.

> **i.** **Benefits:** Improves physical fitness, reduces stress, enhances relaxation, and fosters mental clarity.

3. **Biofeedback:**

> **i.** **Description:** Biofeedback uses electronic monitoring to provide individuals with real-time information about physiological processes like heart rate, muscle tension, or skin temperature. Through this feedback, individuals learn to control these processes.

ii. **Benefits:** Helps manage stress, anxiety, and certain health conditions by improving self-regulation.

4. **Tai Chi:**

i. **Description:** Tai Chi is a Chinese martial art that involves slow, flowing movements, deep breathing, and meditation. It aims to balance the flow of energy (qi) within the body.

ii. **Benefits:** Improves balance, flexibility, and relaxation. It can also reduce stress and enhance mental focus.

5. **Guided Imagery:**

i. **Description:** Guided imagery involves creating mental images to evoke positive sensations and promote relaxation. It often includes visualization exercises led by a practitioner or through recorded scripts.

ii. **Benefits:** Reduces stress, supports emotional well-being, and enhances the mind's ability to influence the body.

6. **Breathwork (Pranayama):**

i. **Description:** Various breathwork techniques, such as deep breathing, diaphragmatic breathing, or alternate nostril breathing, focus on conscious control of the breath to influence mental and physical states.

ii. **Benefits:** Calms the nervous system, reduces stress, and enhances oxygenation of the body.

7. **Progressive Muscle Relaxation (PMR):**

i. **Description:** PMR involves systematically tensing and relaxing different muscle groups to promote relaxation. It heightens awareness of physical sensations and reduces muscle tension.

ii. **Benefits:** Relieves muscle tension, reduces stress, and promotes a sense of calm.

8. **Hypnotherapy:**

i. **Description:** Hypnotherapy uses guided relaxation, focused attention, and suggestion to achieve a heightened state of awareness.

Natural Treatment For Female Infertility

ii. **Benefits:** Addresses various issues, including stress, anxiety, and certain health behaviors, by harnessing the power of suggestion.

9. **Craniosacral Therapy:**

i. **Description:** Craniosacral therapy involves gentle touch and manipulation of the craniosacral system, which includes the skull, spine, and sacrum. It aims to enhance the flow of cerebrospinal fluid and promote overall well-being.

ii. **Benefits:** Supports relaxation, releases tension, and may contribute to emotional balance.

Visualization and Affirmations for Well-Being

1. Visualization Techniques:

i. Guided Imagery: description: Envisioning positive and calming mental images to evoke a sense of peace and well-being.

ii. Process: Close your eyes, relax, and imagine a serene scene, such as a peaceful beach or a tranquil forest.

2.Future Self Visualization:

i. Description: Visualizing your future self in a positive light, achieving goals and living a fulfilling life.

ii. Process: Picture yourself in a successful and content future scenario. Focus on the details of your surroundings, emotions, and accomplishments.

4. Goal Achievement Visualization:

i. Description: Imagining the successful realization of specific goals.

ii. Process: Visualize the step-by-step process of achieving your goals. Picture the challenges, triumphs, and the ultimate accomplishment.

5. Healing Visualization:

i. Description: Using mental imagery to visualize the body's healing process.

ii. Process: Focus on the affected part of the body, visualize it surrounded by healing light or energy. See it becoming healthier and stronger.

6. Affirmation Visualization:

    i. Description: Combining positive affirmations with mental images to reinforce positive beliefs.

    ii. Process: Repeat affirmations while picturing corresponding images. For example, if affirming strength, visualize yourself overcoming challenges.

7. Affirmations:

    i. Positive Self-Affirmations:

    ii. Description: Positive statements that reinforce self-worth and capabilities.

    iii. Examples: "I am confident and capable," "I am deserving of happiness and success," "I am resilient and strong."

8. Fertility Affirmations:

    i. Description: Affirmations focused on promoting a positive mindset during the fertility journey.

    ii. Examples: "My body is strong and capable of creating life," "I trust in my body's natural ability to conceive."

9. Health and Well-Being Affirmations:

    i.   Description: Affirmations centered around maintaining or achieving good health.

10. Mindfulness Affirmations:

i. Description: Affirmations emphasizing present-moment awareness.

ii. Examples: "Try focusing on now (present), and let go of worries and focus on the present."

11. Stress Reduction Affirmations:

i.   Description: Affirmations tailored to alleviate stress and promote relaxation.

Tips for Effective Visualization and Affirmations:

1. Be Specific: Clearly define your visualizations and affirmations to make them more impactful.

2. Use Present Tense: Phrase affirmations as if the desired outcome is already happening.

3. Engage Emotions: Connect emotionally with your visualizations and affirmations to enhance their effectiveness.

4. Consistency is Key: Practice regularly to reinforce positive beliefs and mental images.

5. Combine with Action: Pair visualizations and affirmations with tangible actions that align with your goals.

6. Personalization: Tailor affirmations and visualizations to your unique values, goals, and circumstances.

Remember, the effectiveness of visualization and affirmations can vary from person to person. Consistency and a genuine belief in the process can contribute to their positive impact on mental well-being and overall outlook on life.

CHAPTER SEVEN
Tracking Ovulation And Timing Intercourse

Tracking ovulation and timing intercourse is a common practice for couples trying to conceive. Ovulation is the release of an egg from the ovaries, and it typically occurs in the middle of a woman's menstrual cycle. Here are some methods you can use to track ovulation and optimize the timing of intercourse:

1. **Menstrual Cycle Tracking:** Regular Menstrual Cycle: If a woman has a regular menstrual cycle of 28 days, ovulation is likely to occur around the 14th day. However, this can vary, and cycles can be shorter or longer.

2. **Irregular Menstrual Cycle:** For women with irregular cycles, it can be more challenging to predict ovulation. In such cases, tracking other signs may be more helpful.

3. **Basal Body Temperature (BBT) Charting:** Basal body temperature is the body's resting temperature

and can be measured with a special thermometer. A slight increase in BBT often occurs after ovulation. Tracking this increase over several months can help identify a pattern and predict when ovulation is likely.

4. **Ovulation Predictor Kits (OPKs):** These kits are used to detect surge in the luteinizing hormone (LH) that usually occurs within 24-48 hours before ovulation. When the test indicates a positive result, it's a good time to plan intercourse.

5. **Ovulation Calendar and Apps:** Many smartphone apps and online tools can help you track your menstrual cycle and predict ovulation based on your input.

6. **Regular Intercourse:** Instead of relying solely on pinpointing ovulation, some couples find success by having regular intercourse throughout the menstrual cycle to increase the chances of sperm being present when ovulation occurs.

Remember that these methods are not foolproof, and individual variations exist. Additionally, factors such as

Natural Treatment For Female Infertility

stress, illness, or changes in routine can affect menstrual cycles. If you're having difficulties conceiving, it's advisable to consult with a healthcare professional or a fertility specialist for personalized advice and guidance.

Ovulation Prediction

Ovulation prediction involves identifying the fertile window during a woman's menstrual cycle when ovulation is most likely to occur. Here are some methods used for ovulation prediction:

1. **Basal Body Temperature (BBT) Charting:** Charting basal body temperature involves taking your temperature at the same time every morning before getting out of bed. A slight increase in temperature after ovulation can help pinpoint when ovulation has occurred. However, this method confirms ovulation after it has happened.

2. **Ovulation Predictor Kits (OPKs):** This flow activates the release of egg from the ovary and when the test line is as dark or darker than the control line,

it indicates a positive result and suggests that ovulation is likely to occur soon.

3. **Cervical Mucus Monitoring:** Changes in cervical mucus can indicate fertility. Monitoring these changes can help predict when ovulation is approaching.

4. **Menstrual Cycle Tracking:** For women with regular menstrual cycles, ovulation typically occurs around the middle of the cycle. Tracking the length of your menstrual cycles can provide a rough estimate of when ovulation is likely to occur.

5. **Ovulation Calendar and Apps:** Various smartphone apps and online tools can help you track your menstrual cycle, input symptoms, and predict ovulation based on the information you provide.

6. **Hypothermal Method:** This method combines various signs of fertility, such as BBT, cervical mucus, and cervical position, to predict ovulation more accurately.

It's important to note that these methods have their

Natural Treatment For Female Infertility

limitations, and individual variations exist. Factors such as stress, illness, or changes in routine can affect menstrual cycles and ovulation. Combining multiple methods or consulting with a healthcare professional or fertility specialist can provide a more comprehensive approach to ovulation prediction. Additionally, if you are experiencing difficulties conceiving, it's advisable to seek medical advice for personalized guidance and evaluation.

The Best Times for Conception

The best times for conception, often referred to as the fertile window, center around the woman's ovulation period. Ovulation is the release of an egg from the ovary, and it typically occurs approximately 14 days before the start of the next menstrual period. Here are some key points about the best times for conception:

1. **Ovulation Period:** The most fertile days in a woman's menstrual cycle are the days leading up to, and including, the day of ovulation. For women with regular 28-day menstrual cycles, ovulation is often

around the 14th day. However, it can vary, so tracking signs of ovulation is beneficial.

2. **Fertile Window:** The fertile window is generally considered to be the five days leading up to ovulation and the day of ovulation itself.

3. **Ovulation Predictor Kits (OPKs):** These kits are used to detect the surge in the hormone called the luteinizing hormone (LH) that pave the way for ovulation. Having intercourse during the 24-48 hours after a positive OPK result increases the chances of conception.

4. **Basal Body Temperature (BBT):** Charting basal body temperature can help identify the day of ovulation. A slight increase in temperature after ovulation is an indicator. However, this method confirms ovulation after it has occurred.

5. **Regular Intercourse:** Some couples opt for regular intercourse throughout the menstrual cycle to ensure sperm is present during the fertile window.

6. **Healthy Lifestyle:** Maintaining a healthy lifestyle, including a balanced diet, regular exercise, and managing stress, can positively impact fertility for both partners.

It's important to note that while these methods can improve the chances of conception, they do not guarantee success. Many couples take several months to conceive even when timing intercourse optimally. If you have concerns or if conception is taking longer than expected, consulting with a healthcare professional or a fertility specialist is recommended for personalized advice and evaluation.

Fertility Awareness Methods

Fertility Awareness Methods (FAM) involve tracking various physiological signs and changes in a woman's body to identify fertile and infertile phases of her menstrual cycle. These methods are used for family planning, whether to achieve or avoid pregnancy. Here are key components of Fertility Awareness Methods:

1. **Basal Body Temperature (BBT) Charting: How It**

Natural Treatment For Female Infertility

a. Works: Basal body temperature is the body's resting temperature. A woman's BBT tends to rise slightly after ovulation.

b. Method: Measure your temperature every morning at the same time before getting out of bed. A rise in temperature over several days indicates that ovulation has likely occurred.

c.   **Use:** It helps identify the post-ovulatory infertile phase of the menstrual cycle.

2. **Cervical Mucus Monitoring:**

a. **How It Works:** Changes in cervical mucus consistency can indicate fertility. Around ovulation, mucus becomes clear, slippery, and stretchy, resembling egg whites, creating a hospitable environment for sperm.

b. **Method:** Regularly observe and note changes in the appearance and feel of cervical mucus.

c. **Use:** Identifies the fertile window and helps time intercourse for conception or avoid it for contraception.

3. **Ovulation Predictor Kits (OPKs):**

a. **How It Works:** OPKs detect the surge in luteinizing hormone (LH) that precedes ovulation.

b. **Method:** Use urine tests to identify the LH surge, indicating that ovulation is likely to occur in the next 24-48 hours.

c. **Use:** Pinpoints the fertile window for conception.

4. **Standard Days Method:**

a. **How It Works:** Suitable for women with regular menstrual cycles (26 to 32 days). Avoid intercourse or use contraception on days 8-19 of the menstrual cycle.

Natural Treatment For Female Infertility

b. **Method:** Track your menstrual cycle days and avoid intercourse or use protection during the identified fertile window.

c. **Use:** A simple method for those with regular cycles who want to avoid hormonal contraception.

5. **Symptothermal Method:**

a. **How It Works:** Combines multiple signs such as BBT, cervical mucus, and calendar tracking for a more comprehensive approach.

b. **Method:** Track and interpret various fertility signs concurrently for increased accuracy.

c. **Use:** Offers a more thorough understanding of the menstrual cycle, suitable for both achieving and avoiding pregnancy.

While Fertility Awareness Methods can be effective, they require consistent and accurate tracking. Education and training are crucial for successful implementation. It's also important to note that FAMs are more effective when used

Natural Treatment For Female Infertility

by individuals or couples with regular menstrual cycles and a high level of commitment to tracking and interpreting the signs. If used incorrectly or inconsistently, there is a risk of unintended pregnancies. Couples considering FAMs should consult with a healthcare professional or a fertility educator for guidance.

CHAPTER EIGHT
Fertility Treatments: When Natural Isn't Enough

When natural conception methods are not successful, individuals or couples may explore fertility treatments to assist in achieving pregnancy. Several fertility treatments are available, and the choice depends on the underlying causes of infertility. Here are some common fertility treatments:

1. Fertility Medications:

i. Clomiphene Citrate (Clomid): Stimulates ovulation in women by regulating hormones.

ii. Letrozole: Similar to Clomid, it stimulates ovulation and is sometimes used as an alternative.

2. **In Vitro Fertilization (IVF):** In Vitro Fertilization (IVF) is an assisted reproductive technology that involves the fertilization of an egg with sperm outside the body, in a laboratory setting. This process is used to treat infertility when other methods of assisted

reproductive technologies have not been successful or are not suitable for the couple.

a. **Ovarian Stimulation:** Hormonal injections, such as follicle-stimulating hormone (FSH) and luteinizing hormone (LH), are commonly used.

b. Regular monitoring through blood tests and ultrasound is conducted to track the development of follicles.

3. **Egg Retrieval:** Once the follicles are mature, a minor surgical procedure called egg retrieval or follicular aspiration is performed.

4. **Embryo Transfer:**

   i. **Cryopreservation (Optional):** Any additional viable embryos not transferred may be cryopreserved (frozen) for future use.

5. **Pregnancy Test:** Approximately 10 to 14 days after embryo transfer, a pregnancy test is conducted to determine if implantation has occurred.

IVF is mostly used to tackle the following:

Natural Treatment For Female Infertility

i. Blocked or damaged fallopian tubes.

ii. Unexplained infertility.

iii. Endometriosis.

iv. Ovulatory disorders.

v. Genetic disorders.

While IVF is a highly effective fertility treatment, it may require multiple cycles for success. Success rates vary depending on factors such as the woman's age, the cause of infertility, and the clinic's expertise.

It's important for individuals or couples considering IVF to undergo a thorough evaluation by a fertility specialist. The specialist can provide personalized guidance, discuss potential risks and benefits, and help determine if IVF is the most suitable option for their specific situation. The emotional and financial aspects of IVF should also be carefully considered.

6. **Intrauterine Insemination (IUI):** Intrauterine Insemination (IUI) is often used as a less invasive and more cost-effective option before resorting to more

complex treatments like in vitro fertilization (IVF). Here is an overview of the IUI process:

a. **Ovulation Stimulation:** The woman may be given fertility medications, such as oral medications (like Clomid) or injectable hormones (gonadotropins), to stimulate the ovaries and promote the development of multiple follicles.

b. **Monitoring Ovulation:** Ultrasound monitoring and blood tests are conducted to track the development of follicles and determine the optimal time for ovulation.

c. **Sperm Preparation:** The male partner or a sperm donor provides a sperm sample, which is then processed in the laboratory to concentrate and prepare the healthiest sperm for insemination.

d. **Insemination:** During a woman's fertile window, the processed sperm is introduced directly into the uterus through the cervix using a thin catheter.

e. **Post-Insemination Monitoring:** Some clinics recommend avoiding heavy physical activity for the rest of the day. In some cases, hormonal support, such as progesterone supplements, may be prescribed to support the early stages of pregnancy.

f. **Pregnancy Test:** A pregnancy test is performed around two weeks after the IUI to determine if conception has occurred.

Intrauterine insemination is a treatment that is used commonly for the following situations:

i. Unexplained infertility.

ii. Mild male factor infertility.

iii. Cervical mucus problems.

iv. Couples with a known sperm issue, such as low sperm count or motility.

v. Donor sperm insemination.

While IUI is less invasive and less expensive than IVF, its success rates can vary and depend on factors such as the cause of infertility, the woman's age, and the overall health of both partners. Some couples may need multiple IUI cycles to achieve a successful pregnancy.

It's essential for individuals or couples considering IUI to undergo a comprehensive evaluation by a fertility specialist. The specialist can provide guidance on whether IUI is a suitable option based on the specific circumstances. If IUI is not successful after several attempts, the couple and their healthcare provider may explore other fertility treatment options, such as IVF.

7. **Donor Eggs and Sperm:** Donor eggs and sperm are options for individuals or couples facing infertility issues or those with a higher risk of passing on genetic disorders. These assisted reproductive technologies involve using reproductive cells from a third party to achieve pregnancy. Here's an overview of the processes involving donor eggs and sperm

i. **Egg Donor Selection:** Egg donors are carefully screened for physical health, psychological well-being, and genetic history. Donors may be anonymous or known to the recipients, depending on legal and personal preferences.

iii. **Egg Donor Stimulation:** The egg donor undergoes ovarian stimulation with hormones to produce multiple eggs.

iv. **Egg Retrieval:** The eggs are aspirated from the donor's ovaries using a thin needle.

v. **Fertilization:** The retrieved eggs are fertilized with the male partner's sperm or donor sperm in a laboratory setting through in vitro fertilization (IVF).

vi. **Embryo Transfer:** Healthy embryos resulting from fertilization are transferred into the uterus of the woman who will carry the pregnancy.

vii. **Cryopreservation (Optional):** This is optional because additional embryos must be cryopreserved to be used in the futuree.

8. **Donor Sperm:**

i. **Sperm Donor Selection:** Sperm donors undergo thorough screening for infectious diseases, genetic disorders, and psychological health. Donors may be anonymous or known, depending on regulations and individual preferences.

9. **Sperm Collection and Processing:** The sperm donor provides a semen sample, which is processed in the laboratory to concentrate and prepare the healthiest sperm for fertilization.

10. **Fertilization:** The processed sperm is used for various assisted reproductive techniques, such as intrauterine insemination (IUI) or in vitro fertilization (IVF).

11. **Embryo Transfer or Insemination:** If using IVF, fertilized eggs are transferred into the uterus. If using IUI, the prepared sperm is directly introduced into the woman's uterus.

12. **Considerations: Legal and Ethical Considerations:** Laws and regulations regarding donor eggs and sperm vary by country and region. **Emotional and Psychological Impact:** Using donor eggs or sperm can have emotional and psychological implications. Counseling and support services are often recommended for individuals and couples.

Success Rates: Success rates with donor eggs or sperm can be influenced by various factors, including the age and health of the recipient.

Before choosing donor eggs or sperm, individuals or couples should consult with a fertility specialist to discuss their specific situation, understand the legal and emotional aspects, and explore the best options for achieving a successful pregnancy.

What Is Surrogacy?

Surrogacy: Surrogacy is a reproductive arrangement where a woman, known as a surrogate, carries and gives birth to a baby on behalf of another individual or couple. Surrogacy is an option for individuals or couples who are unable to conceive or carry a pregnancy to term. There are different types of surrogacy arrangements, and the process can involve various legal, ethical, and emotional considerations. Here's an overview of surrogacy:

Types of Surrogacies:

1. **Traditional Surrogacy:** The donor or father of the surrogacy's sperm is usually used to fertilized the egg through artificial insemination.

2. **Gestational Surrogacy:** The embryo is created through in vitro fertilization (IVF), using the egg and sperm of the intended parents or donors.

Process of Surrogacy:

1. **Choosing a Surrogate:** The intended parents may choose a surrogate through agencies, personal connections, or online platforms. Surrogates are typically screened for physical health, psychological well-being, and suitability for surrogacy.

2. **Legal Agreements:** Legal agreements are crucial to outline the rights, responsibilities, and expectations of all parties involved. These agreements often cover issues such as compensation, medical decisions, and custody.

3. **Medical Procedures:** If using gestational surrogacy, the intended mother's eggs or a donor's eggs are fertilized with the intended father's sperm or donor sperm through IVF.

4. **Pregnancy and Birth:** The intended parents are usually present for the birth, and they assume legal custody of the child immediately after birth.

5. **Considerations:**

a. **Legal and Regulatory Issues:** Laws related to surrogacy vary widely by country and even within different states or regions. It's essential to navigate and comply with applicable laws and regulations.

b. **Financial Considerations:** Surrogacy can be expensive, involving costs such as medical procedures, legal fees, and compensation for the surrogate. Honestly, no one is to get involved with surrogacy without knowing the financial implications.

c. **Ethical Considerations:** Ethical concerns may arise related to issues such as compensation, the selection of surrogates, and the potential for exploitation.

Natural Treatment For Female Infertility

> Ensuring the well-being and rights of all parties is essential.

Surrogacy can be a fulfilling option for those struggling with infertility, same-sex couples, or individuals who cannot carry a pregnancy. It's a deeply personal decision, and individuals or couples considering surrogacy should seek legal and medical advice and carefully weigh the emotional, ethical, and financial aspects involved.

Coping With Infertility And Emotional Support

Dealing with infertility can be emotionally challenging for individuals and couples. The journey is often filled with uncertainty, disappointment, and stress. Here are some strategies for coping with infertility and seeking emotional support:

1. Acknowledge and Express Your Feelings: Allow yourself to feel a range of emotions, including sadness, frustration, anger, and grief. It's important to recognize and express these feelings rather than bottling them up.

2. Communicate with Your Partner: It's very crucial for

you to share your fears, thoughts, and hopes with your partner.

3. Seek Professional Counseling: Individual or couples counseling can provide a safe space to discuss emotions and explore coping strategies. A mental health professional experienced in fertility issues can offer guidance and support.

4. Join Support Groups: try as much as possible to join any group that can help support you to have that sense of community and understanding.

5. Educate Yourself: Learn about the various fertility treatments, their success rates, and potential challenges. Understanding the process can help reduce anxiety and empower you to make informed decisions.

6. Set Realistic Expectations: Not every fertility treatment cycle will result in success, and it's okay to acknowledge that.

7. Take Breaks When Needed: You can take breaks if needed. Focus on self-care, hobbies, and activities that bring you joy.

8. Explore Alternative Paths to Parenthood: Be open to exploring alternative paths to parenthood, such as adoption or surrogacy. Understanding and accepting different possibilities can help you navigate your journey.

9. Maintain a Healthy Lifestyle: Pay attention to your physical well-being. A healthy lifestyle, including regular exercise, a balanced diet, and sufficient sleep, can positively impact your emotional state.

10. Limit Stressors: Identify and limit stressors in your life that are unrelated to fertility.

11. Set Boundaries: It's okay to set boundaries regarding discussions about fertility with friends and family.

12. Consider Professional Help for Decision-Making: Fertility specialists and reproductive endocrinologists can provide guidance on treatment options, success rates, and help you make decisions that align with your goals.

Remember that everyone's journey is unique, and there is no one-size-fits-all solution. It's essential to prioritize your emotional well-being and seek the support you need. If you find that your emotional distress is overwhelming, don't hesitate to reach out to mental health professionals who specialize in fertility-related issues.

Dealing with Grief and Loss

Dealing with grief and loss is a complex and individual process that can be challenging and emotionally overwhelming. Whether you're mourning the loss of a loved one, coping with a breakup, facing a health diagnosis, or navigating the emotional impact of infertility or failed attempts at conception, consider doing the following:

1. Acknowledge Your Feelings: Allow yourself to feel a range of emotions, including sadness, anger, guilt, or confusion. It's okay to experience a mix of emotions during the grieving process.

2. Give Yourself Permission to Grieve: Give yourself the time and space to grieve without judgment or pressure.

3. Express Your Emotions: Find healthy ways to express your feelings. This might include talking to a friend, family member, therapist, or writing in a journal. Creative outlets like art or music can also be helpful.

4. Seek Support: Sharing your feelings with others can provide comfort and understanding.

5. Create Rituals: Establishing rituals or ceremonies to honor and remember what or who you've lost can be a meaningful way to cope with grief.

6. Take Care of Yourself:

7. Accept Your Grief Journey: Understand that grief is a non-linear process with no fixed timeline. Be patient with yourself and recognize that healing occurs gradually.

8. Set Boundaries: Be mindful of your emotional limits and communicate your needs to others. It's okay to set boundaries and take time for yourself when necessary.

9. Memorialize and Celebrate: Find ways to celebrate and remember the positive aspects of what or who you've lost. This might involve creating a memorial, establishing a charitable contribution, or continuing a cherished tradition.

10. Explore Spiritual or Faith-Based Support: If spirituality or faith is a part of your life, consider seeking support from your religious community or engaging in spiritual practices that bring comfort.

11. Professional Help: If grief becomes overwhelming or interferes with daily functioning, seeking help from a mental health professional, such as a counselor or therapist, can provide additional support.

12. Educate Yourself on Grief: Understanding the stages and manifestations of grief can help normalize your experiences. There are many resources and books available that explore grief from various perspectives.

Remember that healing from grief is a unique process, and there is no "right" way to grieve. Be compassionate with yourself, and know that seeking support is a sign of strength. If you find that your grief is impacting your daily life or mental health, professional help can offer valuable guidance and support.

Seeking Support

Seeking support is a crucial step in coping with various life challenges, especially in issues pertaining to infertility and childbearing. Here are some avenues for seeking support:

1. Friends and Family: Sometimes, having a supportive

network can provide comfort and understanding.

2. Professional Counselors or Therapists: Mental health professionals, such as counselors, psychologists, or therapists, offer confidential and non-judgmental support. They can help you navigate and cope with various challenges.

3. Support Groups: Joining support groups, whether in person or online, can connect you with others who are going through similar experiences

4. Religious or Spiritual Leaders: Seek guidance and support from religious or spiritual leaders within your community. They often provide emotional support and may offer counseling services.

5. Healthcare Professionals: For physical health challenges or concerns, consult with healthcare professionals who can provide medical advice and support.

6. Hotlines and Helplines: Many helplines and hotlines offer immediate support and a listening ear. These services are often anonymous and can be beneficial in times of crisis.

7. Employee Assistance Programs (EAP): If you're facing

challenges related to work, your employer's EAP can provide confidential counseling services and support.

8. Online Forums and Communities: Participate in online forums or communities where individuals share their experiences and offer support.

9. School Counselors or Advisors: If you're a student, school counselors or advisors can offer guidance and support for academic and personal challenges.

10. Community Centers and Nonprofit Organizations: Local community centers and nonprofit organizations often provide resources and support services. They may offer counseling, workshops, or other forms of assistance.

11. Self-Help Books and Resources: Explore self-help books and resources that provide guidance on coping with specific challenges. Many books offer practical advice and coping strategies.

12. Peer Support Programs: Some organizations have peer support programs where individuals with shared experiences provide support to each other. This can be especially valuable for issues like addiction recovery.

13. Apps and Online Platforms: There are various apps and online platforms designed to offer mental health support, including meditation and mindfulness apps.

14. Legal and Financial Advisors: If you're dealing with legal or financial challenges, seeking advice from professionals in these fields can provide valuable support.

Remember that seeking support is a sign of strength, and there are various resources available to help you through difficult times. Choose the option that feels most comfortable and appropriate for your specific situation. If you're unsure where to start, consider reaching out to a primary care physician, who can provide guidance and referrals to appropriate services.

CHAPTER NINE
Success Stories And Real-Life Experiences

While success stories and real-life experiences can be inspiring, it's essential to approach natural treatments for infertility with an understanding that individual experiences vary. The effectiveness of natural treatments can depend on the specific causes of infertility, and what works for one person may not work for another. Additionally, success stories should not replace professional medical advice or treatment.

That said, some individuals have reported success with certain lifestyle changes and natural approaches to enhance fertility. Here are a few general strategies that some people have found beneficial:

1. **Diet and Nutrition:** Some individuals have reported success with diets rich in antioxidants, vitamins, and minerals. Specific nutrients like folic acid, zinc, and omega-3 fatty acids may play a role in fertility.

2. **Maintaining a Healthy Weight:**Achieving and maintaining a healthy weight through proper diet and

regular exercise may improve fertility for some individuals.

3. **Reducing Stress:** Techniques such as yoga, meditation, and mindfulness may help reduce stress levels.

4. **Regular Exercise:** Engaging in regular, moderate exercise can contribute to overall health, including reproductive health.

5. **Herbal Supplements:** Some individuals explore the use of herbal supplements, such as Vitex (chaste tree), Maca root, or red clover, which are believed by some to have positive effects on hormonal balance and fertility. However, scientific evidence supporting their efficacy is limited, and caution is advised.

6. **Acupuncture and Traditional Chinese Medicine:** Acupuncture and other traditional Chinese medicine practices have been used by some individuals to support fertility. Some studies suggest potential benefits, although more research is needed.

7. **Cycle Tracking and Natural Family Planning:** Monitoring menstrual cycles, basal body temperature, and cervical mucus changes through natural family planning methods may help individuals understand their fertility patterns and identify the fertile window for conception.

It's important to note that these approaches might not address underlying medical issues causing infertility, and they may not be effective for everyone. If you are experiencing infertility and considering natural treatments, it's crucial to consult with a healthcare professional or a reproductive endocrinologist. They can conduct a thorough evaluation, identify potential causes of infertility, and guide you on the most appropriate and evidence-based treatment options for your specific situation. Natural treatments can complement medical interventions, but they should be approached with caution and under professional guidance.

Personal Journeys to Conception

Personal journeys to conception can vary widely, as each individual or couple's experience with fertility is unique.

Natural Treatment For Female Infertility

Here are a few illustrative scenarios that highlight the diversity of paths people may take:

Scenario 1: Natural Conception Success

Couple A:

- **Background:** A healthy, young couple in their 20s decides to start a family.

- **Experience:** After a few months of trying to conceive naturally, the couple successfully becomes pregnant.

- **Outcome:** A healthy pregnancy and the birth of a baby without the need for fertility treatments.

Scenario 2: Fertility Challenges and Medical Intervention

Couple B:

- **Background:** A couple in their early 30s experiences difficulty conceiving after a year of trying.

- **Experience:** Seeking medical advice, they undergo fertility testing, revealing a male factor infertility issue.

Natural Treatment For Female Infertility

- **Treatment:** The couple decides to pursue intrauterine insemination (IUI) with sperm provided by the male partner after appropriate medical interventions.

- **Outcome:** Successful IUI results in pregnancy, leading to the birth of a healthy baby.

Scenario 3: In Vitro Fertilization (IVF) Journey

Individual C:

- **Background:** A woman in her late 30s faces challenges conceiving due to polycystic ovary syndrome (PCOS).

- **Experience:** After several unsuccessful attempts at natural conception, she decides to explore IVF.

- **Treatment:** Undergoing IVF with hormonal stimulation, egg retrieval, and embryo transfer.

- **Outcome:** Successful IVF cycle leads to pregnancy and the birth of a baby.

Scenario 4: Adoption Journey

Couple D:

- **Background:** A couple in their 40s experiences infertility challenges and is unable to conceive despite fertility treatments.

- **Experience:** After exploring various options, they decide to pursue adoption.

- **Process:** Navigating the adoption process, including home studies, legal procedures, and waiting for a match.

- **Outcome:** Adoption brings a child into their lives, and the couple experiences the joy of parenthood.

Scenario 5: Surrogacy Experience

Individual E:

- **Background:** A woman in her 30s faces health issues preventing her from carrying a pregnancy.

- **Experience:** After considering various options, she decides to pursue surrogacy.

- **Process:** Finding a surrogate, legal agreements, and undergoing in vitro fertilization with the help of a surrogate.

- **Outcome:** Successful surrogacy journey results in the birth of a baby, fulfilling the woman's dream of becoming a mother.

These scenarios highlight the diversity of paths individuals and couples may take on their journey to conception. The experiences can involve a range of emotions, decisions, and medical interventions, and each person's story is shaped by their unique circumstances and choices. It's important for individuals and couples facing fertility challenges to seek support, whether from healthcare professionals, support groups, or loved ones, to navigate the emotional and physical aspects of their journey.

Lessons and Inspiration from Others

When it comes to the natural treatment journey for infertility, many individuals and couples have shared their experiences, lessons, and inspiration. While each person's path is unique, there are some common themes that emerge from these stories:

1. **Holistic Health Approach:** Many individuals emphasize the importance of adopting a holistic approach to health, including changes in diet, exercise, and lifestyle. This includes focusing on overall well-being, stress reduction, and maintaining a healthy weight.

2. **Patience and Perseverance:** Natural treatments often require time and patience. Many individuals share the lesson of perseverance, emphasizing the importance of staying committed to lifestyle changes and natural methods even when results may not be immediate.

3. **Mind-Body Connection:** Stories often highlight the mind-body connection and the impact of stress on fertility. Practices such as meditation, yoga, and mindfulness are frequently mentioned as tools for reducing stress and enhancing the chances of conception.

4. **Individualized Approaches:** Many stories emphasize the importance of understanding one's

unique body and fertility challenges. Tailoring natural treatments to individual needs can be a key aspect of success.

5. **Educational Empowerment:** Individuals often stress the importance of educating themselves about fertility, understanding their menstrual cycles, and recognizing signs of ovulation. This knowledge empowers them to make informed decisions about timing and lifestyle changes.

6. **Support Systems:** Building a support system is crucial. Many individuals find strength in connecting with others who are on a similar journey, whether through support groups, online forums, or personal networks. Sharing experiences and advice can be immensely beneficial.

7. **Celebrating Small Victories:** The journey to natural conception can involve ups and downs. Celebrating small victories, whether it's a positive change in health or progress in fertility charting, can help maintain a positive outlook.

8. **Professional Guidance:** Seeking guidance from holistic practitioners, naturopaths, or fertility specialists who support natural approaches is a common theme. Many individuals find value in combining natural treatments with professional advice.

9. **Emotional Well-Being:** Emotional health is integral to the fertility journey. Some stories highlight the importance of addressing emotional aspects, whether through counseling, journaling, or other forms of self-care.

10. **Maintaining Hope and Optimism:** Despite challenges, maintaining hope and optimism is a recurring theme. Many individuals share stories of unexpected success after periods of doubt, reinforcing the idea that the fertility journey can be unpredictable.

11. **Flexibility in Approach:** Being flexible and willing to adjust strategies is a lesson echoed in many stories. If one approach doesn't yield results, individuals

Natural Treatment For Female Infertility

often explore other natural treatments or consider a
combination of approaches.

It's important to note that natural treatments may not be
suitable for everyone, and individual experiences can vary
widely. Before embarking on any fertility journey,
consulting with healthcare professionals or fertility
specialists is recommended to ensure a comprehensive
understanding of one's unique situation and to receive
personalized guidance.

About The Book

"Natural Treatment for Female Infertility" is a step-by-step guide written by Mrs. Vera Jacob because of the hundreds of millions of women who have lost hope of experiencing the joy of motherhood, women who are scared of leaving their matrimonial home because they thought they could not conceived, women who have suffered countless miscarriages, and who are suffering from fertility-related issues like; ovulation diseases, PCOS, POI, endometriosis, uterine fibroid, hormonal imbalance and lots more.

This guide explores alternative and holistic approaches to addressing infertility in women and provides insights on evidence-based information, and practical advice on natural treatments that would aid in enhancing fertility, understanding how factors like environmental influences, nutrition, stress, and emotional well-being can impact fertility, the underlying causes of infertility, and discussing lifestyle modifications, dietary considerations, different natural remedies and practices that can prevent, intervene and treat infertility, empowering women to make informed decisions and take an active role in their fertility journey.

www.ingramcontent.com/pod-product-compliance
Lightning Source LLC
Chambersburg PA
CBHW070906260726
48661CB00004B/1621